First Edition
First Printing 2018

In the U. S. write to purchase copies:
Datcajungirlprecious@gmail.com

©Copyright 2017
Precious Place Accessories
& More, LLC
All Rights Reserved
Printed in USA

Cover Design:
Designs With Rhythm

Edited By:
Designs With Rhythm

Train Your Brain and Reign

My Testimony...

I had a fight with Fibromyalgia and I WON...One of the many challenges I faced was medicine induced mental illness, delayed brain response and memory loss. The Power of God's Word ZAPPED my Brain and Restored my life. Restoration is yours, wherever you are in life.

Welcome to the New you...through a 21 day Daily Devotional

Train Your Brain and Reign

MIND RENEWED

~NOTES~

Train Your Brain and Reign

Day 1- My Mind Renewed

Today's Scripture

"Be ye transformed by the renewing of your mind"

(Romans 12:2)

A Prayer for Today

Father God in the Name of Jesus. I am clothed in My right Mind and My mind is renewed day by day in the Name of Jesus. Amen

~NOTES~

Train Your Brain and Reign

VICTORY

~NOTES~

DAY 2- My Complete Victory

Today's Scripture

"Being confident of this, that he who began a good work in you will carry it on to completion until the day of Christ Jesus."
(Philippians 1:6, NIV)

A Prayer for Today

Father God in the Name of Jesus. I am confident that the Good work You started in my Life, You are Man enough to Complete it. I go forth into this day knowing that I have Complete victory in the name of Jesus. Amen

~NOTES~

Train Your Brain and Reign

STIR IT UP

~NOTES~

DAY 3- My Preparation for Manifestation

Today's Scripture

Jesus replied, Truly I tell you, if you have faith and do not doubt, not only can you do what was done to the fig tree, but also you can say to this mountain, Go, throw yourself into the sea and it will be done (Matthew 21:21, NIV)

A Prayer for Today

Heavenly Father, thank You for Your Word which is life to ignite my mind, I receive Your strength today to run over troops and leap over walls. Power is in my mouth to speak faith filled words. Thank You for preparing a path of victory as I keep my heart and mind pure and stayed on You in Jesus' name. Amen

Train Your Brain and Reign

~NOTES~

REMEMBER

Train Your Brain and Reign

~NOTES~

DAY 4- My One Day at a Time

Today's Scripture
"Remember the wondrous works that he has done, his miracles, and the judgments he uttered."

(Psalm 105:5, ESV)

A Prayer for Today

Father God, right now I take time to remember and acknowledge Your goodness, grace, and mercy in my life. I praise You because You are good. Thank You for loving me. Thank You for setting me free. Thank You for the outpouring of Your blessings on me and leading me into everlasting life in Jesus' name. Amen.

Train Your Brain and Reign

~NOTES~

GOD KNOWS

Train Your Brain and Reign

~NOTES~

DAY 5- My Grace to Maintain

Today's Scripture

"...Neither do I concern myself with great matters, nor with things too profound for me."
(Psalm 131:1, NKJV)

A Prayer for Today

Father, today I surrender my questions; I surrender my past; I know You will tell me the things I need to know on a need to know basis. I surrender my need to have all the answers. Today I choose to trust You with my life. I keep focused in Jesus' name. Amen.

Train Your Brain and Reign

~NOTES~

I AM ANOINTED

Train Your Brain and Reign

~NOTES~

DAY 6- Another Chance For Me

"...For God has appointed another seed for me..."

(Genesis 4:25, NKJV)

A Prayer for Today

Father God, you are the giver of all life! You give life to all my dreams and visions. You give life to all my relationships, and life to my mind, body, and soul.

Today I choose to release myself into my destiny and embrace the gift of life You have in store for my future.

I am determined to go all the way with You in Jesus' name. Amen.

Train Your Brain and Reign

~NOTES~

A NEW HEART

Train Your Brain and Reign

~NOTES~

DAY 7 - My Total Restoration

Today's Scripture

"In their hearts humans plan their course, but the LORD establishes their steps."
(Proverbs 16:9, NIV)

A Prayer for Today

Heavenly Father, I submit my mind, will and heart to You. I am sick and tired of making mistakes. Help me to see clearly what Your plan is for me. Help me to stay close to You always, not living in defeat but pressing forward to the new things You have in store for me as I purge my heart in Jesus' name. Amen.

Train Your Brain and Reign

~NOTES~

NEW MERCIES

Train Your Brain and Reign

~NOTES~

DAY 8 - A Whole New Beginning for Me

Today's Scripture

"It is of the Lord's mercies that we are not consumed, because his compassion fails not. They are new every morning: great is thy faithfulness
(Proverbs 16:9, NIV)

A Prayer for Today

Heavenly Father, I am so grateful for Your love. Today I get another chance. Thank You for an outpouring of Your mercy upon my life. Lord give me the Power to help others by telling my story for God's glory in Jesus' name. Amen.

Train Your Brain and Reign

~NOTES~

GOD'S GLORY

Train Your Brain and Reign

~NOTES~

DAY 9 - My Manifestation Time

Today's Scripture

"For our light and momentary troubles are achieving for us an eternal glory that far outweighs them all."

(2 Corinthians 4:17, NIV)

A Prayer for Today

Heavenly Father, thank You for working Your manifested glory in me. I cast my every care on You, knowing that my trials and troubles are temporary. My appointed time is near. Thank You for Your kingdom blessing on my life today and always in Jesus name. Amen

Train Your Brain and Reign

~NOTES~

I AM PLANTED

Train Your Brain and Reign

~NOTES~

DAY 10- I Shall Not Be Moved

Today's Scripture

"He will be like a tree firmly planted by streams of water, which yields its fruit in its season and its leaf does not wither; and in whatever he does, he prospers."

(Psalm 1:3, NASB)

A Prayer for Today

Father God, I love You so much today. Thank You for Your Word which is truth and hydration to my soul. Search me, know me, and guide me in the way that I should go as I stay unshakable in you and planted in Your Word. I shall not be uprooted in Jesus name. Amen

Train Your Brain and Reign

~NOTES~

I AM THE LIGHT

Train Your Brain and Reign

~NOTES~

DAY 11- Jesus Comes To My Rescue

Today's Scripture

"When darkness overtakes him, light will come bursting in..."

(Psalm 112:4, TLB)

A Prayer for Today

Heavenly Father, thank You for Your light that drives out every mark of darkness! I am expecting signs, wonders, and miracles to follow my life. I choose to focus on Your faithfulness. I am fully persuaded You are working behind the scenes, and I expect that You will turn things around for me. I give you Praise in Advance in Jesus Mighty name. Amen.

Train Your Brain and Reign

~NOTES~

Train Your Brain and Reign

I AM FILLED

~NOTES~

DAY 12- God Is Alive in Me

Today's Scripture

"And if the Spirit of him who raised Jesus from the dead is living in you, he who raised Christ from the dead will also give life to your mortal bodies because of his Spirit who lives in you." (Romans 8:11, NIV)

A Prayer for Today

Father in heaven, thank You for filling me with Your power by the Holy Spirit. I choose to fuel my faith by declaring Your Word. I choose to walk in Your ways and honor You in everything I do and say. My kingdom integrity is grafted in me in Jesus' name. Amen.

~NOTES~

Train Your Brain and Reign

BE STRONG

~NOTES~

Train Your Brain and Reign

DAY 13- I Choose to Believe

Today's Scripture

"And David said to his son Solomon, 'Be strong and of good courage, and do it; do not fear nor be dismayed, for the LORD God--my God--will be with you. He will not leave you nor forsake you, until you have finished all the work for the service of the house of the LORD'."
(1 Chronicles 28:20, NKJV)

A Prayer for Today

Father God, I choose to believe in Your Word, even when things look impossible. I choose to believe that You are working behind the scenes and that You will bring victory and breakthrough to every area of my life in Jesus' name. Amen.

~NOTES~

Train Your Brain and Reign

I AM WITH YOU

~NOTES~

Train Your Brain and Reign

DAY 14- No Fear Lives Here

Today's Scripture

"Be strong and courageous. Do not be frightened, and do not be dismayed, for the LORD your God is with you wherever you go."
(Joshua 1:9, ESV)

A Prayer for Today

Heavenly Father, thank You for loving me in spite of me Thank You for Your faithfulness. I know that You are amazing, and you are closer to me than the air I breathe. Today I receive Your promises in faith and choose to cast all my cares on You in Jesus' name. Amen.

~NOTES~

Train Your Brain and Reign

AWESOME GOD

~NOTES~

DAY 15- My End Shall be Greater

Today's Scripture

"Declaring the end from the beginning, and from ancient times things that are not yet done..."

(Isaiah 46:10, NKJV)

A Prayer for Today

Father God, how awesome You are! Thank You for declaring, decreeing, and praying over my Life. I choose to Speak Your Word, even when I don't understand. I trust that You are good and that my end shall be greater than my beginning in Jesus' name! Amen.

~NOTES~

Train Your Brain and Reign

I AM HIS

~NOTES~

Train Your Brain and Reign

DAY 16- I Am Full of Favor

Today's Scripture

"Keep me as the apple of your eye..."
(Psalm 17:8, NIV)

A Prayer for Today

Father in heaven, thank You for kissing my day with opportunity. Thank You for keeping me the apple of Your eye. I open my heart and mind to You. I am a genius and a money absorber. I receive Your love for me in Jesus' name. Amen.

~NOTES~

Train Your Brain and Reign

BE THANKFUL

~NOTES~

Train Your Brain and Reign

DAY 17- I Follow My Leader

Today's Scripture

"But thanks be to God, Who in Christ always leads us in triumph..."
(2 Corinthians 2:14, AMP)

A Prayer for Today

Heavenly Father, I come to You with genuine sincerity and right motives. God, I have your intentions. I thank You for the victory that You have in store for my Pastor. Make me one with my leader. I choose not to frustrate him or her, but, instead I will be an extension of him or her in Jesus' name. Amen

~NOTES~

Train Your Brain and Reign

ARISE

~NOTES~

DAY 18- This is My Set Time

Today's Scripture

"You will arise and have mercy on Zion; for the time to favor her, yes, the set time, has come."

(Psalm 102:13, NKJV)

A Prayer for Today

Father God, thank You for this day. Thank You for the good plan You have for me. I believe it is my time of set favor; it's my time to rise higher; it's my time to experience every breakthrough and every blessing You have in store for me in Jesus' name! Amen.

~NOTES~

Train Your Brain and Reign

COMEBACK POWER

~NOTES~

DAY 19- My Multiplied Grace Activated

Today's Scripture

"He gives power to the weak, and to those who have no might He increases strength."
(Isaiah 40:29, NKJV)

A Prayer for Today

Heavenly Father, thank You for Your favor, strength, and grace at work in my life. I turn my focus on You today. I turn my thoughts on You. I set my heart and love upon You because You are good. Thank You for filling me with might and power to overcome in Jesus' name! Amen.

~NOTES~

Train Your Brain and Reign

NO LIMITS

~NOTES~

Train Your Brain and Reign

Day 20- My Peace

Today's Scripture

"I have seen that everything [human] has its limits and end [no matter how extensive, noble, and excellent]; but Your commandment is exceedingly broad and extends without limits [into eternity]." (Psalm 119:96, AMPC)

A Prayer for Today

Father in heaven, today I lift my eyes to You. You alone are the source of my strength, peace, and provision. I choose to delight myself in You knowing that You will give me the desires of my heart in Jesus' name. Amen.

~NOTES~

Train Your Brain and Reign

SILENCE NO MORE

~NOTES~

Train Your Brain and Reign

Day 21- Lord Fill Me Again

Today's Scripture

"Open your mouth wide, and I will fill it..."
(Psalm 81:10, NLT)

A Prayer for Today

Heavenly Father, I come to you today asking you to fill me again . I choose to trust You even when I don't understand how everything is going to work out. I know you are a good God. I am full of patience and I humbly wait on You. My Mouth will only speak those things from your word In Jesus Name Amen

~NOTES~

Train Your Brain and Reign

ABOUT THE AUTHOR

Lisa has been caring for people for over 33 years as a nurse and a servant.

Founder of Precious Signature Seasonings/(DaBayou Cajun Seasoning) Local and Global supplier for Walmart, other local businesses such as Brookshire's and Drug Emporium enjoys cooking, hospitality, and serving. She is also the author of 2 other Books: *"DaBayou Cajun Recipe Cookbook"* and *"I Gotta' Throw Myself Into the Ministry Servant's Handbook."*

www.ingramcontent.com/pod-product-compliance
Lightning Source LLC
Chambersburg PA
CBHW070311230526
45470CB00002B/823